SYSTEM INNOVATION

Disruptor Diary

SYSTEM INNOVATION

Disruptor Diary

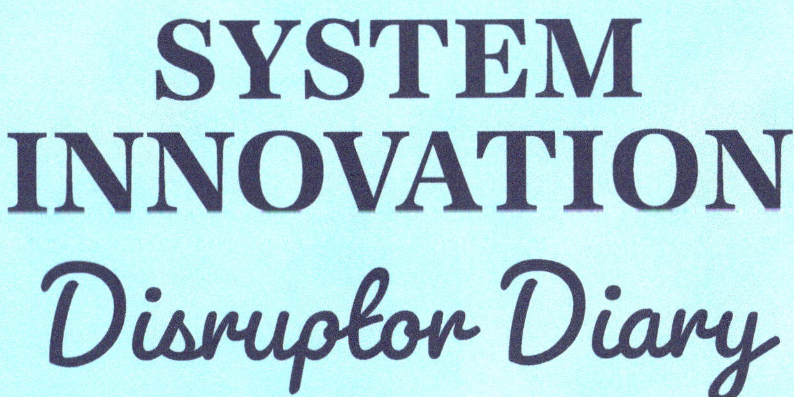

A Holistic Approach to Disrupting with Love and Human Caring

Julie Kennedy Oehlert and
Kathleen Sitzman

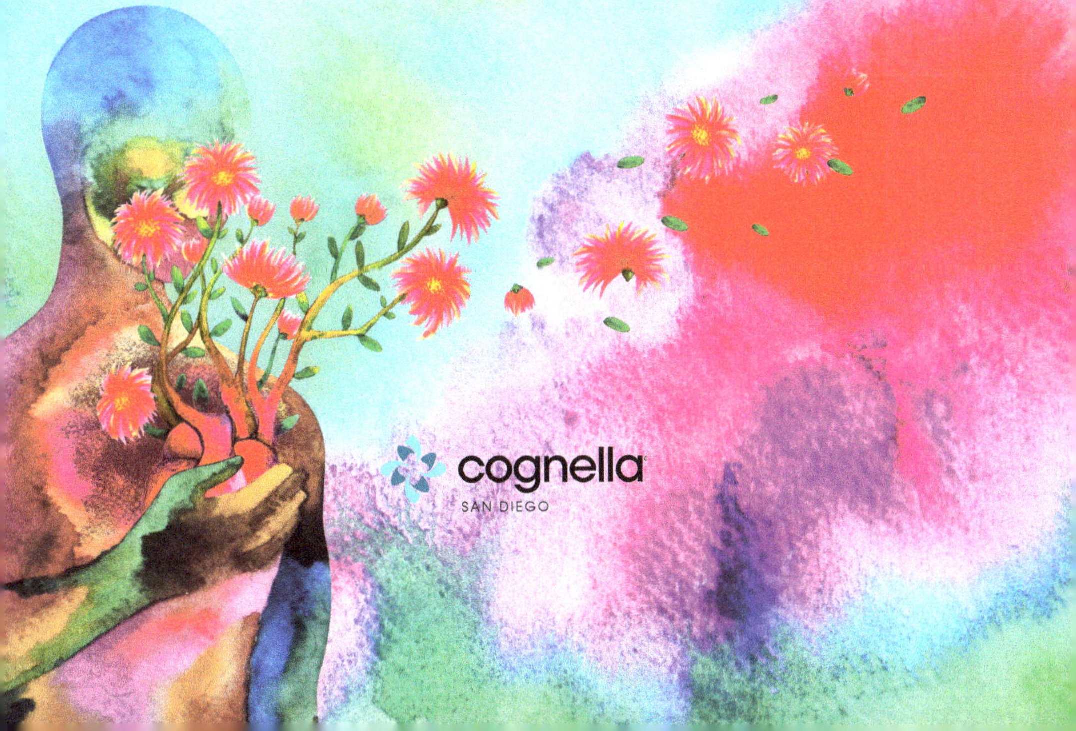

cognella
SAN DIEGO

Bassim Hamadeh, CEO and Publisher
Amanda Martin, Executive Publisher
Amy Smith, Associate Editorial Manager
Jeanine Rees, Production Editor
Jess Estrella, Senior Graphic Designer
Kylie Bartolome, Licensing Specialist
Natalie Piccotti, Director of Marketing
Kassie Graves, Senior Vice President, Editorial

Printed in the United States of America.

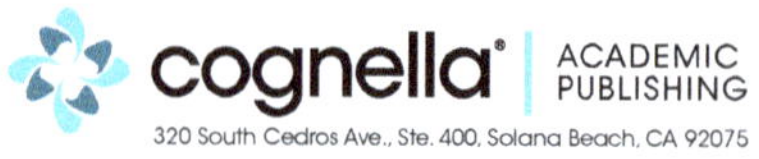

Note from the Authors

This disruptor diary was designed for you to use with the book *System Innovation: A Holistic Approach to Disrupting with Love and Human Caring*, which lays out a foundational, holistic approach for facilitating successful disruption at the healthcare system level. It shares theoretic models and conceptual frameworks, as well as implementable operational concepts and practices. Our hope is that our book stimulates readers to advance disruption within healthcare organizations so that a more beautiful, loving, and caring healthcare system can emerge.

This disruptor diary celebrates and affirms you as an important disruptor by providing the space for reflection, journaling, and ideation, in honor of how vital the thoughts and ideas of healthcare workers are to its very future.

We have collected some of our favorite quotes from each chapter, and provided additional space for you to further reflect, doodle, journal, and engage.

We have also included two impactful exercises from Chapters 2 and 7 of System Innovation; one on designing your own disruption mandala, and the other, a deep reflection on customer service versus hospitality.

We hope you spend time with each chapter of System Innovation and reflect on how your own ideas, innovations, and musings can be a disruptive force to improve healthcare for all through the lens of love and human caring.

—Julie Kennedy Oehlert, DNP, RN
—Kathleen Sitzman, PhD, RN, CNE, ANEF, FAAN

CHAPTER 1

Innovation and Theory

Authors' note: We love how theory expands our thinking and provides scaffolding for disruption in so many ways!

Theories help challenge and expand what is possible, and innovate beyond what is probable.

> *There is a key concept to the idea of disruption: the understanding that cultures may maintain or transform based on the relational interactions of those within the culture.*

Cultures do not get 'fixed' or 'changed' but transform themselves through the structure of all the relational disruption and silos.

CHAPTER 2

Silos and Disruption

When we think of healthcare system innovations, we reflect on silos and the exciting possibilities imaginable if those silos were dismantled and new power with transpersonal caring relationships were fostered to unite the separated entities.

When the fundamental concepts, approaches and assumptions of an industry change, this is called disruptive change. Once the shift has occurred, the system rarely returns to its previous state (Potter, 2022).

Sample Mandala

The beauty of the Disruption Mandala is that it is customizable. In its beauty and balance it reminds us all that disruption does not have to be destructive or ugly—it can be beautiful, transformative, and uplifting and lead to an upward spiral of innovations of higher achievement, especially when infused with generous amounts of love and human caring.

We invite you to spend some time creating your own system Disruption Mandala by reflecting on what departments or areas you would identify as siloed and would benefit from system innovations using a holistic approach to disrupting with love and human caring.

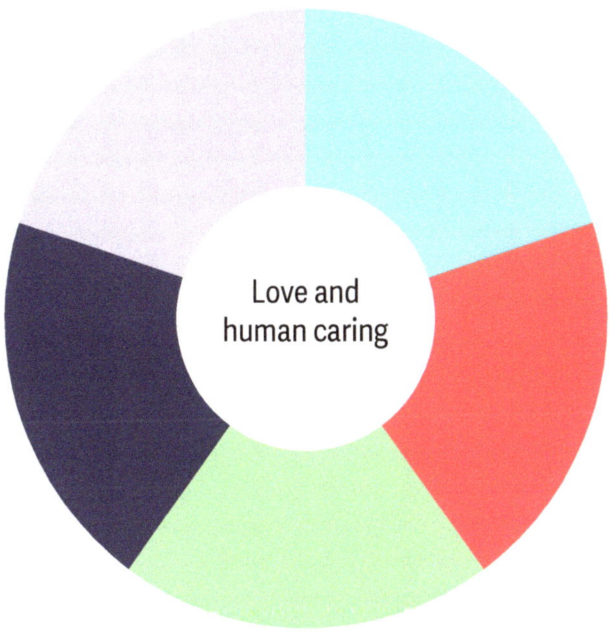

FIGURE 2.1 Blank Disruption Mandala

CHAPTER 3

Leadership Is Love

Leadership is in the driver's seat when it comes to culture. Culture eats strategy for breakfast, and leaders are the ones cooking that breakfast and serving it up.

It can be a wholehearted revelation in leadership development for leaders to work on their capacity for love or human caring to become a more effective leader.

Leadership is not power over, *it is the* power with *and the power to create caring environments through love.*

Healthcare is not transactional, it is relational.

CHAPTER 4

Measurement

Goal-Setting for Love and Human Caring

Data is powerful. Data can inspire and invigorate or it can demean and disengage.

Encouraging and rewarding the culture to focus on the positives—creating more loving or caring interactions—versus the negatives will help the environment stay out of a punitive power over mindset.

Go towards what you want,
not away from what you don't!

A score card cannot coach, interpret, encourage, or reward, only a loving, caring and wise leader can do that.

CHAPTER 5

Human Resources Transformation

Human Resources is the marketing department for team members.

Attracting talent, versus "recruiting" talent sets the tone for a humanistic process that begins from the first contact with the organization, when potential new hires are getting to know the culture of the organization.

Policies within an organization have the power to hold a culture in place despite desired disruption if they are not reviewed and adapted to the current or desired culture on a regular basis.

CHAPTER 6

Organizational Communication

Listen to and Connect With Each Other

Organizations can solve every problem encountered, past, present and future, by asking their team members for solutions.

Effective communication in organizations is both a science and an art, and requires deliberate prioritization and commitment to listen to all of the humans in the organization in an ongoing flow of ideas, experiences, and insights.

Multidimensional caring communication supports power with environments and enables trust, authentic presence, full listening, and mindful consideration of both positive and negative feelings.

CHAPTER 7

Human Caring Experience

The New Hospitality

You will not punish people into loving.

Healthcare is not transactional but rather a series of connected transpersonal power with relationships that should benefit those who receive care as well as those who provide care.

Patient experience is a manifestation of team engagement and well-being. Taking care of each other and our teams equals taking care of our patients and families.

Review the definitions of customer service and hospitality in the visual below. Reflect on each definition, and how they may or may not support and advance Cultural Transformation Theory power with relationships and Watson's Ten Caritas Processes®.

Service	Hospitality
• The technical delivery	• The feeling imparted
• Monologue	• Dialogue
• Standardized	• Personalized, customized
• To people	• With people
• The "what"	• The "how"

FIGURE 7.1 Hospitality vs. Customer Service.

Watson's Ten Caritas Processes®

- Embrace altruistic values and practice lovingkindness with self and others.
- Be authentically present, enable faith and hope, and honor others.
- Be sensitive to self and others by nurturing individual beliefs and practices.
- Develop helping-trusting-caring relationships.
- Promote and accept positive and negative feelings as you authentically listen to another's story.
- Use creative scientific problem-solving methods for caring decision-making and creative solution-seeking.

(Adapted from The Experience Lab LLC, "Hospitality vs. Customer Service, Watson's 10 Caritas Processes®." Copyright © by The Experience Lab LLC. Reprinted with permission.)

CHAPTER 8

Healthcare Voices

Catalysts for Disruption

Innovation is often the light shining from the hearts of those in the middle of disaster, providing inspiration, hope and ultimately paves a new, better path forward.

Authors' Note: We put in your hands the future of healthcare as a loving and human caring profession. We thank you for your engagement in *System Innovations: A Holistic Approach to Disrupting with Love and Human Caring*.

—Julie Kennedy Oehlert, DNP, RN
—Kathleen Sitzman, PhD, RN, CNE, ANEF, FAAN

www.ingramcontent.com/pod-product-compliance
Ingram Content Group UK Ltd.
Pitfield, Milton Keynes, MK11 3LW, UK
UKHW021829270726
14058UKWH00001B/49